Energy Healing Through Reiki:

WORKBOOK EXERCISES

*supplementary book for note-taking
and practice session recording*

By Melissa Crowhurst

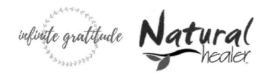

Contents

Completing the exercises...4

Remember the "5 Reiki Principles".................................5

Practice the "Hand Energy Exercise" 6

Practice "Determining Your Power Hand" 7

Practice "Letting Go" 8

Practice "Intentions"...9

Practice "Protection" 10

Practice "Spiritual Detox" 11

Practice "Reiki Symbols" (Draw & Activate) 12

Practice "Chakras" 17

Practice "Scanning"...19

Practice "Healing Attunements" 20

Practice "Traditional Reiki Hand Positions" 23

Practice "Distance Attunements" 25

Requesting Your Certificate 27

Completing the exercises

Throughout the *Energy Healing Through Reiki - Reiki Master Course* handbook and lectures, there are various reminders, such as the "**Workbook Exercise: Practice!**" sections in the handbook, which prompt you to come here to complete the relevant exercises.

When that happens, simply go to the appropriate section of this workbook and practice the exercise, then record your findings and make appropriate notes.

Whenever you see "☐ **Practice Session 1 | ☐ Practice Session 2 | ☐ Practice Session 3**", the numbers are simply there to indicate the number of times you practice. So in the example above, you practice 3 times. Simply tick the boxes as you complete your practice sessions.

Once you complete a workbook session, enter the date (DD/MM/YY) which you completed the section.

This workbook is for your own reference, it acts as a place to keep track of your practice sessions as well as log your own feelings and notes. I suggest you keep this workbook handy when taking your final exam, too – as it will help you with providing correct answers ☺

Lastly, please remember that your journey to mastery is about taking your time to embrace the lesson and practice, so you truly connect with that Universal Life Force Energy – so please don't rush this process – and always follow your heart! Okay, are you ready? Let's begin!

Remember the "5 Reiki Principles"

After you've taken the time to read the principles to yourself in Chapter 1, list out all *Five Reiki Precepts* here:

1. _____

2. _____

3. _____

4. _____

5. _____

6. Do you think you'll be able to include these precepts into your way of life? Explain here:

_____

Date completed: _____

Practice the "Hand Energy Exercise"

After you've taken the time to review the steps on how to *feel Reiki* in Chapter 2; now practice the exercise several more times.

This can be done in one sitting, or over a period of time, it's up to you.

☐ Practice Session 1

☐ Practice Session 2

☐ Practice Session 3

Did you notice any difference in the feeling of energy between your first try and the last session? List out any observations you felt during your practice sessions:

_____

_____

_____

_____

Date completed: _____

Practice "Determining Your Power Hand"

Perform the *Hand Energy Exercise* a few times and while you go through the process, assess:

- Which hand seems stronger in sensation?
- Has one has become more tingly than the other?
- Perhaps one is very cold or extremely hot?

Note down your observations, as well as which hand you think your Power Hand may be:

_____

_____

_____

_____

Date completed: _____

Practice "Letting Go"

After reading about "Letting Go" in Chapter 3; take some time to practice doing it with the exercise below:

I'd like you to think about an event in your life that's recently happened where the outcome wasn't what you wanted.

For example, an anticipated trip was cancelled due to bad weather; you had an argument during a dinner that was meant to be romantic; or you got caught in a traffic jam which made you late for work...

How does that memory make you feel now?

If you feel anything other than calm, content or happy – then you probably need to practice the art of "letting go" – which is effectively you *removing your expectation* on any outcome.

Meditation is a great way to learn how to "let go". So if you haven't already, you're welcome to listen to a variety of free meditations on my YouTube channel here: https://www.youtube.com/c/NaturalhealerAu

You may also want to read or listen to my blog post for more tips on letting go http://naturalhealer.com.au/2016/06/truly-forgive/

Record any notable feelings or thoughts about this exercise here:

_____

_____

Date completed: _____

Practice "Intentions"

After you've taken the time to review the steps on how to *set intentions* in Chapter 3; now practice the exercise several more times.

This can be done in one sitting, or over a period of time, it's up to you.

☐ Practice Session 1

☐ Practice Session 2

☐ Practice Session 3

Did setting intentions become progressively easier as you moved from your first try to the last session?   Record down any notes or observations from your practice sessions:

_____

_____

_____

Date completed: _____

Practice "Protection"

After you've taken the time to review the steps on *protection methods* in Chapter 3; now practice them several more times.

This can be done in one sitting, or over a period of time, it's up to you.

☐ Practice Visualization 1

☐ Practice Visualization 2

☐ Practice Visualization 3

Did you find it easy to visualize the protection methods? Record down any notes or observations from your practice sessions:

_____

_____

_____

Date completed: _____

Practice "Spiritual Detox"

In Chapter 3, I discuss "spiritual detoxing" and making some lifestyle changes to help your healing.

Make a commitment to yourself now, be it short or long term, to make positive adjustments to your lifestyle so you can better help yourself and others.

☐ I have reduced/eliminated: _____

_____

☐ I have increased/added: _____

_____

How does this commitment to your own personal health make you feel?

_____

_____

Date completed: _____

Practice "Reiki Symbols" (Draw & Activate)

In Chapter 4, you learned the Reiki Symbols. I'd like you to now practice drawing them and activating them here to the best of your ability.

Remember, you can simply say the name of the symbol for those more complex ones, until you get the hang of drawing them. This can be done in one sitting, or over a period of time, it's up to you.

1. Cho Ku Rei (Power Symbol)

☐ Practice Drawing 1   ☐ Practice Drawing 2   ☐ Practice Drawing 3

☐ Practice Activation 1 ☐ Practice Activation 2 ☐ Practice Activation 3

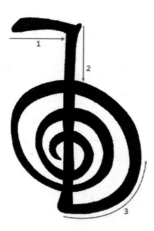

Did you notice any feeling in your hands, or dominant hand, while practicing? Did you notice any energy or feelings change around you?

_____

Date completed:
_____

2. Sei Hei Ki (Emotional Symbol)

☐ Practice Drawing 1   ☐ Practice Drawing 2   ☐ Practice Drawing 3

☐ Practice Activation 1 ☐ Practice Activation 2 ☐ Practice Activation 3

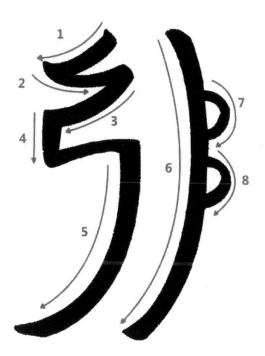

Did you notice any feeling in your hands, or dominant hand, while practicing? Did you notice any energy or feelings change around you?

_____

Date completed: _____

3. Hon Sha Ze Sho Nen (Distance Symbol)

☐ Practice Drawing 1   ☐ Practice Drawing 2   ☐ Practice Drawing 3

☐ Practice Activation 1 ☐ Practice Activation 2 ☐ Practice Activation 3

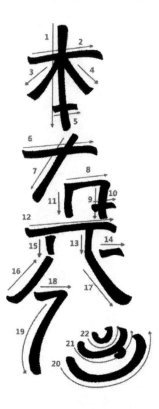

Did you notice any feeling in your hands, or dominant hand, while practicing? Did you notice any energy or feelings change around you?

_____

Date completed:

_____

4. Dai Ko Myo (Usui Master Symbol)

☐ Practice Drawing 1   ☐ Practice Drawing 2   ☐ Practice Drawing 3

☐ Practice Activation 1 ☐ Practice Activation 2 ☐ Practice Activation 3

Did you notice any feeling in your hands, or dominant hand, while practicing? Did you notice any energy or feelings change around you?

_____

Date completed:

5. Raku (Grounding Symbol)

☐ Practice Drawing 1   ☐ Practice Drawing 2   ☐ Practice Drawing 3

☐ Practice Activation 1 ☐ Practice Activation 2 ☐ Practice Activation 3

Did you notice any feeling in your hands, or dominant hand, while practicing? Did you notice any energy or feelings change around you?

_____

Date completed: _____

Practice "Chakras"

Because the form of Reiki you're learning revolves around Chakra positioning – it's important you know where they are on the body.

Do you remember what "Chakras" are, and what their purpose is in the body?

_____

_____

_____

How does Reiki affect the "Chakras"?

_____

_____

Referring to the chart on the next page, on the appropriate lines, list out the corresponding Chakra (a) names and (b) colours - from memory:

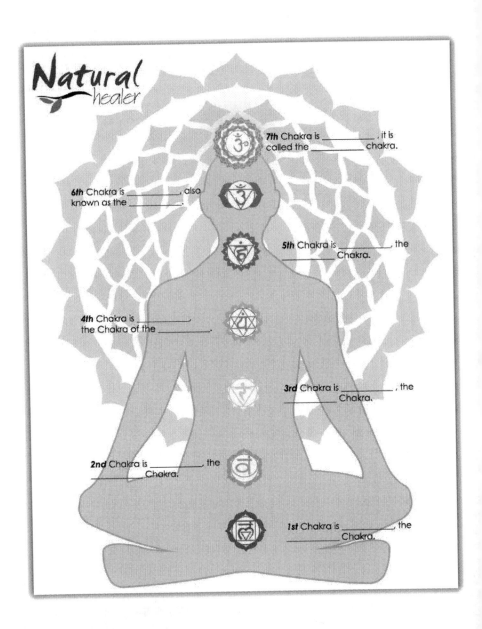

Natural healer

7th Chakra is _____ , it is called the _____ chakra.

6th Chakra is _____ , also known as the _____ .

5th Chakra is _____ , the _____ Chakra.

4th Chakra is _____ , the Chakra of the _____ .

3rd Chakra is _____ , the _____ Chakra.

2nd Chakra is _____ , the _____ Chakra.

1st Chakra is _____ , the _____ Chakra.

Date completed: _____

18

Practice "Scanning"

In Chapter 6, you learn how to "scan" yourself and others. To get the hang of it, perform scanning sessions on yourself, as well as others (don't forget, you can perform some sessions on an animal or object).

Don't try and do this is all in one sitting, space your scanning sessions out.

☐ Practice Self Scan 1

☐ Practice Self Scan 2

☐ Practice Self Scan 3

How did you feel before, during, and after your own scanning sessions?

_____

☐ Practice Scan on Others 1

☐ Practice Scan on Others 2

☐ Practice Scan on Others 3

How did you feel before, during, and after the scanning sessions? Did your client feel or notice anything?

_____

Date completed: _____

Practice "Healing Attunements"

In Chapter 7, you learn how to perform a healing "attunement". To get the hang of it, perform sessions on yourself, as well as others (don't forget, you can perform some sessions on an animal or object).

Self-healing – please don't try and do this is all in one sitting, space your healing sessions out.

☐ Practice Self-Healing Attunement 1

☐ Practice Self-Healing Attunement 2

☐ Practice Self-Healing Attunement 3

Now please complete 30 self-healings to ensure you remain balanced and attuned to the *Universal Life Force Energy* – please don't try to do this all in one sitting, please space these sessions out.

☐ 1 ☐ 2 ☐ 3 ☐ 4 ☐ 5 ☐ 6 ☐ 7 ☐ 8 ☐ 9 ☐ 10

☐ 11 ☐ 12 ☐ 13 ☐ 14 ☐ 15 ☐ 16 ☐ 17 ☐ 18 ☐ 19 ☐ 20

☐ 21 ☐ 22 ☐ 23 ☐ 24 ☐ 25 ☐ 26 ☐ 27 ☐ 28 ☐ 29 ☐ 30

How did you feel before, during and after your self-healings?

_____

_____

Date completed: _____

General Healing – please don't try and do this is all in one sitting, space your healing sessions out.

☐ Practice General Healing Attunement (Person) 1

☐ Practice General Healing Attunement (Person) 2

☐ Practice General Healing Attunement (Person) 3

☐ Practice General Healing Attunement (Person) 4

☐ Practice General Healing Attunement (Person, Animal or Object) 5

How did you feel before, during, and after the attunement? Did your attunee feel or notice anything?

_____

_____

_____

Date completed:

_____

Specific Healing – please don't try and do this is all in one sitting, space your healing sessions out.

☐ Practice Specific Attunement (Person) 1

☐ Practice Specific Attunement (Person) 2

☐ Practice Specific Attunement (Person) 3

☐ Practice Specific Attunement (Person) 4

☐ Practice Specific Attunement (Person, Animal or Object) 5

How did you feel before, during, and after the attunement? Did your attunee feel or notice anything?

_____

_____

_____

Date completed: _____

Practice "Traditional Reiki Hand Positions"

Also in Chapter 7, you learned the "Traditional Reiki Hand Positions" both for healing others and for self-healing. To get the hang of it, perform sessions on yourself, as well as others (don't forget, you can perform some sessions on an animal or object).

Traditional Reiki Hand Positions (Self-Healing) – please don't try and do this is all in one sitting, space your sessions out.

☐ Practice Traditional Reiki Hand Positions – Self-healing 1

☐ Practice Traditional Reiki Hand Positions – Self-healing 2

☐ Practice Traditional Reiki Hand Positions – Self-healing 3

How did you feel before, during, and after the session?

_____

_____

_____

Date completed: _____

Traditional Reiki Hand Positions (On Others) – please don't try and do this is all in one sitting, space your sessions out.

☐ Practice Traditional Reiki Hand Positions (Person) 1

☐ Practice Traditional Reiki Hand Positions (Person) 2

☐ Practice Traditional Reiki Hand Positions (Person) 3

☐ Practice Traditional Reiki Hand Positions (Person) 4

☐ Practice Traditional Reiki Hand Positions (Person, Animal or Object) 5

How did you feel before, during, and after the session?

_____

_____

_____

Date completed: _____

Practice "Distance Attunements"

In Chapter 7, you learn how to perform a "distance attunement". To get the hang of it, perform sessions on yourself, as well as others (don't forget, you can perform some sessions on an animal or object).

General Distance Healing – please don't try and do this is all in one sitting, space your healing sessions out.

☐ Practice General Healing Distance Attunement (Person) 1

☐ Practice General Healing Distance Attunement (Person) 2

☐ Practice General Healing Distance Attunement (Person) 3

☐ Practice General Healing Distance Attunement (Person) 4

☐ Practice General Healing Distance Attunement (Person, Animal or Object) 5

How did you feel before, during, and after the attunement?

_____

_____

_____

Date completed: _____

Specific Distance Healing – please don't try and do this is all in one sitting, space your healing sessions out.

☐ Practice Specific Healing Distance Attunement (Person) 1

☐ Practice Specific Healing Distance Attunement (Person) 2

☐ Practice Specific Healing Distance Attunement (Person) 3

☐ Practice Specific Healing Distance Attunement (Person) 4

☐ Practice Specific Healing Distance Attunement (Person, Animal or Object) 5

How did you feel before, during, and after the attunement? Did your attune feel or notice anything?

_____

_____

_____

Date completed: _____

Requesting Your Certificate

Once you've completed this workbook and all the lectures of the course 100%, you'll be ready to complete your final exam, and then request for your certificate.

You will gain access to the certificate request form link once you've completed all the course lectures 100% - so please refer to the course lectures further information.

Please note, I manually review each certificate request, so to avoid delays, please ensure you have done all the steps in the course – including having your Reiki Student Attunement Ceremony done by me, complete your self-healings, do your practice sessions, pass your final exam, as well as have fully read and understood all the course material – <u>before</u> you request your certificate.

If you have any questions about this process, please ask me or my support team by logging into your student account.

Thank you, it's been an honour! From here on out, I hope you continue to shine your light my sweet friend and fellow healer. #biglove

Ways to connect with Melissa:

Melissa's Blog

https://naturalhealer.com.au/blog/

Facebook

https://www.facebook.com/naturalhealerau

YouTube

https://www.youtube.com/c/NaturalhealerAu

ITunes

https://itunes.apple.com/au/podcast/natural-healer/id1133780594?mt=2

Twitter

https://twitter.com/naturalhealerau

Instagram

https://www.instagram.com/naturalhealerau/

Made in the USA
Middletown, DE
01 June 2024

55131274R00018